# Chronic Pain Management

## A Comprehensive Guide to Management and wellness

**Dr. Daniel  Thompson**

# Copyright

No part of this book should be copied ,reproduced without the author's permission © 2023. Chronic Pain Management . Dr. Daniel Thompson.,

# TABLE OF CONTENT

# Chapter 1

# Introduction to Chronic Pain

Chronic pain is a widespread and intricate health problem that affects millions of people globally and goes beyond simple discomfort. This introduction delves into the complex nature of chronic pain, examining its definition, extent, and the wide range of negative effects it has on one's quality of life. Furthermore, we offer a perceptive synopsis of the various chronic pain disorders that people experience, illuminating the complexities of this enduring problem.

## Definition and Scope

To put it simply, chronic pain is any kind of discomfort that lasts longer than the normal course of an injury or disease. In contrast to acute pain, which acts as a defense mechanism and goes away as the injury heals, chronic pain lasts longer,often longer than three to six months. It crosses over into the psychological and social spheres, combining with the physiological, making it a difficult and complicated condition to treat completely.
The term "chronic pain" refers to a wide range of conditions, including neuropathic, musculoskeletal, inflammatory, and psychogenic pain. Its influence extends beyond age, gender, and socioeconomic status, impacting people from all backgrounds. From the persistent ache of arthritis to the stabbing sensations of

neuropathy, chronic pain manifests in various forms, defying a one-size-fits-all approach to understanding and managing its complexities.

## The Impact on Quality of Life

Chronic pain is more than just a feeling; it's a force that can change a person's life and affect every part of their being. Its effects extend well beyond the physical, impacting social interactions, emotional health, and general quality of life. Constant pain can cause a variety of negative effects, such as mood swings, sleep disturbances, and a decreased ability to perform daily tasks.

People who deal with chronic pain frequently have to navigate a maze of difficulties. Easy chores become difficult, relationships may suffer as a result of the illness, and it may become difficult to work or engage in hobbies. The significant negative influence on quality of life highlights the need for all-encompassing approaches to chronic pain management that take into account not just the physical symptoms but also the emotional and social aspects of the individual's experience.

## Overview of Chronic Pain Conditions

It is important to recognize the variety of conditions that are included under the general category of chronic pain in order to fully understand it. Every illness has different difficulties, signs, and treatment options. For instance, neuropathic pain, which manifests as tingling, burning, or shooting pain, results from injury to or malfunctions in the nervous system. On the other hand, musculoskeletal pain typically affects the tendons, ligaments, muscles, and bones and is brought on by chronic illnesses like fibromyalgia or injuries.

The immune response of the body is connected to inflammatory pain, which results in pain and swelling. The complex relationship between the mind and body in the experience of pain is highlighted by psychogenic pain, which has its origins in emotional or psychological variables.These ailments only make up a small portion of the complex field of chronic pain, highlighting the necessity of individualized and focused strategies to meet the particular difficulties that each presents.

It takes a thorough understanding of chronic pain conditions that extends beyond their physical symptoms to navigate their complexities. It demands an understanding of the psychological cost, the effect on relationships, and the uniqueness of the experience. Through acquiring knowledge about these facets, patients and medical professionals can cooperate to develop efficient chronic pain management plans that improve overall health.

# Chapter 2

# Understanding Types of Chronic Pain

The term "chronic pain" refers to a wide range of conditions that people struggle with on a daily basis and cannot be adequately defined. This chapter delves deeply into the study of four main categories of persistent pain: inflammatory pain, musculoskeletal pain, psychogenic pain, and neuropathic pain. Since each type has different difficulties, managing them effectively and giving affected parties targeted relief requires a sophisticated understanding of these issues.

## Neuropathic Pain

### Definition and Origins:

The cause of neuropathic pain, which is frequently referred to as a difficult and complex condition, is abnormalities in the nervous system. Neuropathic pain develops when the nerves themselves become dysfunctional, in contrast to nociceptive pain, which is caused by tissue injury. A number of things, such as illnesses, injuries, or problems with the central or peripheral nervous systems, can cause this.

## Characteristics and Symptoms:

The distinguishing features of neuropathic pain are its hallmark. People frequently describe experiencing pain that feels electric shock-like, burning, shooting, or tingling. These feelings could come on suddenly or in reaction to non-painful stimuli. One of the most well-known characteristics of neuropathic pain is that it is chronic in nature, meaning it lasts for long periods of time and frequently resists standard pain management techniques.

## Common Causes:

Numerous conditions can cause neuropathic pain, such as peripheral neuropathy, diabetic neuropathy, shingles-related postherpetic neuralgia, and nerve compression syndromes like carpal tunnel syndrome. Neuropathic pain can also be brought on by trauma, infections, and certain medications.

## Diagnosis and Treatment Approaches:

To effectively manage neuropathic pain, an accurate diagnosis is imperative. To find the root cause, doctors frequently use a mix of clinical histories, physical examinations, and diagnostic testing. Once a diagnosis has been made, treatment may take a multimodal approach, including physical therapy, medical interventions like nerve blocks, and medications like anticonvulsants and antidepressants.

# Inflammatory Pain

**Nature and triggers:**

The immune system's reaction to an injury, infection, or illness causes inflammation-related pain in the body. It is a defense system intended to get rid of dangerous stimuli and encourage recovery. But chronic inflammation can cause pain that lasts longer than the original injury or infection, as in the case of rheumatoid arthritis or inflammatory bowel disease.

## Features and Signs:

Localized pain, swelling, redness, and heat in the afflicted area are signs of inflammatory pain. Many people describe the pain as throbbing or aching, and it may also be accompanied by stiffness and a decreased range of motion. Persistent inflammation can exacerbate pain by causing tissue damage.

## Common Reasons:

Irritable bowel diseases (such as Crohn's disease and ulcerative colitis) and chronic inflammatory conditions (such as tendinitis and bursitis) are among the many conditions that are categorized as inflammatory pain. Infections and specific metabolic conditions have been linked to inflammatory pain.

## Methods of Diagnosis and Treatment:

A comprehensive assessment of the patient's clinical symptoms, imaging studies, and laboratory testing to detect inflammatory markers are all necessary for the diagnosis of inflammatory pain. Pain management and inflammation reduction are the goals of treatment plans. In addition to dietary and exercise changes, nonsteroidal anti-inflammatory drugs (NSAIDs), disease-modifying antirheumatic drugs (DMARDs), and corticosteroids are frequently used.

# Musculoskeletal Pain

## Nature and Triggers:

Musculoskeletal pain pertains to discomfort arising from the muscles, bones, ligaments, tendons, and joints. It is a prevalent type of chronic pain, often resulting from trauma, overuse, or underlying chronic conditions affecting the musculoskeletal system.

## Characteristics and Symptoms:

The nature of musculoskeletal pain can vary widely, encompassing dull aches, sharp stabbing sensations, or a persistent throbbing. Pain may be localized to a specific area or radiate along the affected muscle or joint. Individuals often report stiffness, tenderness, and reduced flexibility as accompanying symptoms.

## Common Causes:

Conditions contributing to musculoskeletal pain include osteoarthritis, rheumatoid arthritis, fibromyalgia, myofascial pain syndrome, and traumatic injuries such as fractures or sprains. Additionally, poor ergonomics, sedentary lifestyles, and repetitive strain injuries can contribute to the development of musculoskeletal pain.

## Diagnosis and Treatment Approaches:

Diagnosing musculoskeletal pain involves a combination of clinical evaluation, imaging studies, and, in some cases, laboratory tests. Treatment strategies aim to address the underlying cause, manage symptoms, and improve function. This may include physical therapy, analgesic medications, muscle relaxants, and lifestyle modifications such as regular exercise and proper ergonomics.

# Psychogenic Pain

## Nature and Initiations:

Psychogenic pain is a complicated phenomenon where psychological factors influence how pain is perceived and manifested. It is also known as psychosomatic pain or somatoform pain disorder. Psychogenic pain may not have a definite physical cause, in contrast to other forms of chronic pain.

## Features and Significance:

Headaches, stomachaches, or widespread pain throughout the body are just a few of the symptoms that can indicate psychogenic pain. It is frequently distinguished by a discrepancy between the degree of pain that the patient reports and the lack of physical pathology that can be identified. While the person feeling the pain knows it exists, emotional and psychological factors play a major role in its genesis.

## Common Reasons:

Anxiety disorders, depression, somatization disorders, and unresolved emotional trauma are some of the causes of psychogenic pain. Stressors or emotional disturbances can intensify or initiate psychogenic pain due to the complex mind-body connection.

It takes a thorough assessment by medical professionals, such as doctors and mental health specialists, to diagnose psychogenic pain. The goal is to comprehend the psychological elements influencing the perception of pain. A multidisciplinary approach is frequently used in treatment, combining stress management methods, psychotherapy, cognitive-behavioral therapy (CBT), and, in certain situations, pharmaceuticals.

# Combining Information to Provide Complete Care

Comprehending the subtleties of these forms of chronic pain is crucial for medical practitioners, caregivers, and those who experience the pain. It establishes the foundation for a customized and all-encompassing approach to pain management by realizing that successful tactics go beyond just treating physical symptoms. The development of focused interventions that improve overall well-being is made possible by the recognition of the interactions between biological, psychological, and social factors.

# Chapter 3

# Causes and Risk Factors

Millions of people worldwide suffer from chronic pain, a widespread and complex ailment that reduces quality of life and presents management challenges. Creating comprehensive plans for managing and reducing chronic pain requires an understanding of the complex network of causes and risk factors that contribute to the condition. This chapter explores the complex nature of chronic pain, including the underlying medical conditions, lifestyle factors, genetic predispositions, and environmental influences that all play a significant role in its onset and persistence

## Underlying Medical Conditions

### Role in Chronic Pain:

Underlying medical conditions serve as primary catalysts for the initiation and perpetuation of chronic pain. These conditions span a broad spectrum, ranging from musculoskeletal disorders and neurological conditions to autoimmune diseases and metabolic disorders. The connection between these medical conditions and chronic pain is complex, often involving intricate interactions between physiological pathways and nervous system .

1.Musculoskeletal disorders :
Musculoskeletal disorders such  as osteoarthritis, rheumatoid arthritis, and fibromyalgia are prominent contributors to chronic pain. These disorders involve inflammation, joint degeneration,

and widespread pain, significantly impacting an individual's quality of life.

2. Neurological Conditions:
Neurological disorders, including neuropathies, multiple sclerosis, and migraines, can lead to chronic pain. The damage or dysfunction of the nervous system in these conditions results in altered pain processing, amplifying and prolonging pain sensations.

3.  Autoimmune Diseases:
Autoimmune diseases like lupus and rheumatoid arthritis trigger an immune response against the body's own tissues, causing inflammation and, consequently, chronic pain. The persistent immune activity contributes to long-term discomfort and pain.

4.  Metabolic Disorders:
 Metabolic disorders, such as diabetes, can lead to nerve damage (diabetic neuropathy), contributing to chronic pain. The systemic impact of metabolic imbalances adds a layer of complexity to the pain experience.

## Environmental Factors

### Influence on Chronic Pain:

Environmental factors play a significant role in shaping an individual's experience of chronic pain. These factors encompass the physical, social, and cultural aspects of one's surroundings, influencing pain perception and its impact on daily life.

1. Physical Environment:

Living in environments with excessive noise, pollution, or ergonomic challenges can exacerbate chronic pain. Factors like inadequate lighting and uncomfortable furniture can contribute to physical discomfort and musculoskeletal pain.

2.Social Environment:
The social support network, or lack thereof, can profoundly influence chronic pain. Individuals with strong social connections often experience better emotional well-being, which can positively impact their ability to cope with and manage chronic pain. Conversely, social isolation or strained relationships can contribute to heightened stress and worsened pain outcomes.

3. Cultural Factors:
Cultural beliefs and attitudes toward pain can shape an individual's response to chronic pain. Cultural norms around expressing pain, seeking medical help, and utilizing pain management strategies can vary, influencing an individual's experience and approach to chronic pain.

# Genetic Predisposition

## Genetic Factors in Chronic Pain:

Genetic predisposition plays a crucial role in an individual's susceptibility to chronic pain. Certain genetic variations can influence pain sensitivity, the efficacy of pain medications, and the likelihood of developing specific pain conditions.

1. Pain Sensitivity Genes:
Genes involved in pain processing, such as those related to neurotransmitters and receptors, can influence an individual's pain

sensitivity. Variations in these genes may contribute to heightened or reduced sensitivity to pain stimuli.

2. Pharmacogenetics: Genetic factors also play a role in how individuals respond to pain medications. Variations in genes related to drug metabolism and receptor interactions can impact the effectiveness and side effects of analgesic medications.

3. Inherited Pain Conditions:
Some individuals may inherit conditions that predispose them to chronic pain. Examples include familial pain syndromes and genetic connective tissue disorders, which can influence pain perception and musculoskeletal function.

# Lifestyle Contributors

## Lifestyle Choices and Chronic Pain:

Lifestyle choices, encompassing aspects of daily living such as diet, physical activity, sleep patterns, and stress management, play a pivotal role in the development and management of chronic pain. These contributors are modifiable factors that individuals can address to positively impact their pain exexperience

1.Sedentary Lifestyle:
A lack of physical activity and prolonged periods of sitting or inactivity can contribute to musculoskeletal pain and stiffness. Regular exercise promotes circulation, flexibility, and the release of endorphins, which act as natural pain relievers.

2.Poor Diet:

Nutritional choices can influence inflammation and overall health, impacting chronic pain. Diets high in processed foods, sugar, and saturated fats may contribute to inflammation, exacerbating pain in conditions like arthritis.

3. Sleep Disturbances:
Quality sleep is essential for overall health and plays a crucial role in pain perception. Chronic pain conditions, in turn, can disrupt sleep, creating a cyclical relationship. Addressing sleep disturbances becomes integral to comprehensive pain mamanagement

4.Stress and Emotional Well-being:
Chronic stress and emotional distress contribute to the perpetuation of chronic pain. The mind-body connection is intricate, and stress can exacerbate pain conditions. Techniques such as mindfulness and stress reduction become vital components of pain management ststrategies.

5.Substance Use:
The use of certain substances, including tobacco and excessive alcohol consumption, can negatively impact chronic pain. Nicotine, for example, can affect blood flow and contribute to inflammation, while alcohol can disrupt sleep patterns and exacerbate pain conditions.

# The Interconnected Web of Causation

Understanding chronic pain necessitates recognizing the interconnected web of causation that involves a dynamic interplay between underlying medical conditions, environmental influences, genetic predisposition, and lifestyle contributors. Individuals often experience a combination of these factors, and unraveling this complexity is crucial for tailoring effective and personalized interventions.

## Comprehensive Assessment and Personalized Strategies

Healthcare professionals employ comprehensive assessments to identify the specific causes and risk factors influencing an individual's chronic pain experience. This involves a thorough medical history, diagnostic tests, and consideration of environmental and lifestyle factors. Personalized strategies can then be developed, addressing the unique aspects of each individual's pain profile.

## Empowering Individuals through Knowledge

Empowering individuals with knowledge about the diverse causes and risk factors associated with chronic pain is a crucial step in fostering active participation in their own care. By understanding the multifaceted nature of chronic pain, individuals can make informed choices, collaborate with healthcare providers, and adopt lifestyle modifications that positively impact their pain experience.

# Chapter 4

# Medications and Treatments

Chronic pain management requires a multifaceted approach that integrates various medications and treatment modalities aimed at alleviating discomfort, improving function, and enhancing the overall quality of life for individuals grappling with persistent pain. In this chapter, we explore a spectrum of interventions, ranging from pharmaceuticals to surgical procedures and emerging treatments, each playing a pivotal role in the comprehensive management of chronic pain.

## Analgesics and Anti-Inflammatory Medications

### Role in Pain Management:

Analgesics and anti-inflammatory medications form the cornerstone of pharmacological interventions for chronic pain. These medications serve diverse purposes, aiming to reduce pain intensity, alleviate inflammation, and enhance the individual's ability to engage in daily activities.

1.Nonsteroidal Anti-Inflammatory Drugs (NSAIDs):
NSAIDs, such as ibuprofen and naproxen, work by inhibiting enzymes responsible for inflammation. They are commonly used to manage pain associated with inflammatory conditions like arthritis. However, long-term use of NSAIDs may pose risks of gastrointestinal bleeding and cardiovascular complications.

2. Acetaminophen:
Acetaminophen, while lacking anti-inflammatory properties, functions as a pain reliever and fever reducer. It is frequently utilized for mild to moderate pain management. Caution is advised to avoid exceeding recommended doses due to potential liver toxicity.

3.Opioids:
Opioids, including morphine, oxycodone, and hydrocodone, are potent pain relievers used for severe chronic pain. However, their use is controversial due to the risk of addiction, tolerance, and adverse effects, necessitating careful prescribing and monitoring by healthcare providers.

4. Adjuvant Medications:
Certain medications, initially developed for conditions other than pain, demonstrate efficacy in managing specific chronic pain types. Antidepressants, anticonvulsants, and muscle relaxants are often prescribed as adjuvants to alleviate neuropathic pain or to address associated symptoms like sleep disturbances and mood disorders.

# Physical Therapy

## Role in Pain Rehabilitation:
Physical therapy plays a pivotal role in chronic pain management by focusing on restoring function, reducing pain, and improving overall physical well-being. It encompasses a range of therapeutic exercises, modalities, and interventions tailored to individual needs.

1. Therapeutic Exercise:
Exercise programs designed by physical therapists aim to improve flexibility, strength, and endurance while minimizing pain. These programs may include stretching exercises, low-impact aerobic activities, and resistance training.

2.Manual Therapy:
Manual techniques, such as massage, joint mobilization, and manipulation, are employed to alleviate muscle tension, improve range of motion, and reduce pain. These techniques target specific areas of discomfort, aiding in relaxation and pain relief.

3. Modalities and Interventions:
Physical therapists utilize various modalities, including heat and cold therapy, electrical stimulation, ultrasound, and hydrotherapy, to alleviate pain, reduce inflammation, and promote healing.

# Surgical Interventions

### Considerations for Chronic Pain:

Surgical interventions are considered in specific cases where conservative treatments fail to provide relief or when anatomical abnormalities or injuries necessitate surgical correction. Surgical options for chronic pain vary based on the underlying condition and individual circumstances.

1.Spinal Interventions:
Procedures such as spinal fusion, discectomy, and laminectomy are performed to address spinal conditions causing chronic pain, including herniated discs, spinal stenosis, or vertebral fractures.

These surgeries aim to stabilize the spine or alleviate nerve compression.

2.Joint Replacement: For severe joint degeneration causing chronic pain, joint replacement surgeries like hip or knee replacements are considered. These surgeries aim to restore function, alleviate pain, and improve mobility.
3. Nerve Blocks and Neurostimulation:
Interventional procedures such as nerve blocks and neurostimulation techniques involve the use of injections or implanted devices to disrupt pain signals or modulate nerve activity, providing relief for certain chronic pain conditions like neuropathic pain or complex regional pain syndrome (CRPS).

# Emerging Treatments

## Innovative Approaches in Pain Management:

Advancements in medical research and technology continue to pave the way for novel approaches to chronic pain management. Emerging treatments encompass innovative therapies that hold promise in addressing pain more effectively or targeting specific pain pathways.

1.Regenerative Medicine:
Regenerative therapies, including platelet-rich plasma (PRP) injections and stem cell therapy, aim to promote tissue repair and regeneration, potentially offering relief for conditions involving tissue damage or degeneration.

2. Biofeedback and Virtual Reality:
Technological innovations in biofeedback and virtual reality therapy offer non-invasive approaches to pain management.

These therapies involve training individuals to control physiological functions or immersing them in virtual environments to distract from pain sensations.

3.Targeted Drug Delivery Systems:
Advances in drug delivery systems allow for targeted and localized delivery of medications to specific pain sites. Implantable devices or injectable formulations enable precise administration of medications, reducing systemic side effects.

# Integrating Comprehensive Care

The diversity of medications and treatments available for chronic pain underscores the importance of a multidisciplinary and personalized approach to care. Healthcare providers collaborate to tailor interventions, considering the individual's specific pain profile, underlying conditions, treatment goals, and potential risks associated with each modality.

# Chapter 5

# Lifestyle Modifications for Pain Management

Chronic pain management is more than just medicine; it includes a variety of lifestyle changes that have a big impact on how someone feels about their pain. This chapter examines the role that posture and ergonomics, dietary modifications, stress-reduction strategies, and sleep hygiene play in the efficient management of chronic pain. These lifestyle changes are intended to reduce pain, improve general health, and work in conjunction with other pain management techniques.

## Ergonomics and Posture

### Significance in Pain Control:

A key factor in lowering musculoskeletal strain and easing chronic pain is good posture and ergonomics. The goal of these modifications is to reduce stress on muscles, joints, and ligaments by optimizing the environment and body alignment. This will lessen pain and help to prevent further injuries.

1. Workplace Ergonomics:
For people who spend a lot of time at desks or in front of computers, adjusting workstations to encourage good posture is crucial. This involves placing the keyboard in the right location,

maintaining neutral body alignment, adjusting desks, and using ergonomic chairs in order to lessen strain.

2.Body Mechanics:
Pain levels can be greatly impacted by maintaining appropriate body mechanics when performing daily tasks like lifting heavy objects, bending, or standing for extended periods of time. Methods like lifting using your legs rather than your back and avoiding repeated actions reduce the risk of strain and damage.

3. Posture Awareness:
 By making conscious efforts to keep your back straight when standing, sitting, and walking, you can lessen the strain on your joints and muscles. Ergonomic supports such as footrests or lumbar cushions can help to keep the spine in a neutral alignment and minimize pain.

# Dietary Adjustments

## Effect on Sensation of Pain:

Making dietary changes is essential for controlling inflammation, lessening pain, and enhancing general health. Some foods have anti-inflammatory qualities, but other foods can make inflammation worse, which can affect how someone feels pain.

1. Anti-Inflammatory Diet:
To reduce inflammation, concentrate on eating whole foods high in omega-3 fatty acids, antioxidants, and phytonutrients. To achieve this, consume a diet high in fruits, vegetables, nuts, seeds, fatty fish, and healthy fats like olive oil, and low in processed foods, sugars, and trans fats.

2.Hydration:
 Sustaining tissue health and enabling normal physiological processes require adequate hydration. Maintaining proper hydration can help with pain management by lowering tenseness in the muscles, strengthening joints, and improving general wellbeing.
**Weight Management:** When it comes to managing chronic pain, especially conditions like osteoarthritis or back pain, maintaining a healthy weight is essential. While weight management efforts can reduce strain and discomfort, being overweight places additional stress on joints and tissues.


# Stress Reduction Techniques

## Effect on Sensation of Pain:

There are complex relationships between stress and pain, and controlling stress can have a beneficial impact on how someone feels chronic pain. The main goals of stress reduction techniques are to calm the body and mind, ease emotional distress, and lessen physiological reactions that might make pain worse.

1.Mindfulness and Meditation:
Techniques like guided imagery, deep breathing exercises, and mindfulness-based stress reduction (MBSR) assist people in focusing on the present moment, lowering their anxiety levels, and adjusting how they perceive pain.
#### Relaxation Techniques: Progressive muscle relaxation, yoga, and biofeedback are a few examples of techniques that help people relax, release tension from their muscles, and feel more at ease. These techniques help lessen the discomfort and muscle spasms brought on by chronic pain.

2. Cognitive Behavioral Therapy (CBT):
CBT methods help people recognize and change harmful thought patterns and actions that increase pain and stress. This therapy enhances general mental health and aids in the development of coping skills.

# Sleep Hygiene

## Effects on Suffering and Recuperation:

For the treatment of pain and general health, getting enough sleep is essential. A vicious cycle frequently develops between chronic pain and sleep disturbances, where pain exacerbates poor sleep, which in turn causes more pain. Encouraging restful sleep through the use of good sleep hygiene practices helps manage pain.

1.Ambience for Sleep: Improving elements like lighting, temperature, and mattress comfort as well as reducing noise disturbances are all part of creating a comfortable space for sleeping. More pain relief and higher-quality sleep are encouraged in a cozy sleeping environment.

2. Regular sleep schedule: The body's internal clock is regulated by keeping a regular sleep schedule that includes regular wake-up and bedtime times. By encouraging restorative sleep patterns, this enhances the quality of sleep and helps manage chronic pain.

3.Relaxation Techniques Before Bed: By relaxing the body and mind before bed, you can minimize pain-related disturbances and set yourself up for a restful night's sleep. Some examples of these activities include reading, gentle stretching, or taking a warm bath.

## Including Lifestyle Adjustments

Effective treatment of chronic pain requires incorporating these lifestyle changes into regular activities. To get the most pain relief and overall well-being, people can combine these strategies and customize them to fit their unique needs and preferences.

## A Joint Method for Pain Management

Healthcare professionals are essential in informing people about these lifestyle changes and helping them to be implemented. For these changes to be successfully implemented and maintained, cooperation between healthcare providers, people with chronic pain, and support systems is essential.

# Chapter 6

# Pain Management Techniques

## Mindfulness Practices

Being mindful entails intentionally focusing on the experiences of the present moment while avoiding passing judgment. Mindfulness practices are intended to foster an awareness of pain-related sensations, thoughts, and emotions in the context of managing chronic pain.

## Getting to Know Mindfulness:

People who engage in mindfulness practices learn to view their experiences—including pain—with an accepting and non-reactive mindset. People can develop a sense of detachment from pain-related distress by learning more about their bodies' reactions through practices like focused breathing or body scans.

**1.Aware Mindfulness**
:By acknowledging pain sensations without allowing them to control or define one's entire experience, one can practice mindful awareness. People can lessen the emotional impact of pain by simply observing these sensations without passing judgment.

**2.Mindfulness-Based Stress Reduction (MBSR):**
To reduce stress and pain, MBSR programs combine mindfulness meditation, yoga, and cognitive-behavioral methods. These courses offer methodical direction for integrating mindfulness into day-to-day activities, fostering emotional health and resilience.

**3.Daily Awareness:**

Promoting mindfulness in daily tasks like eating, walking, and even brushing teeth aids people in developing awareness in everyday situations. This encourages the development of a regular mindfulness practice outside of focused sessions

## Meditation Techniques

By refocusing attention, calming the mind, and fostering a sense of calmness, meditation can help manage the emotional distress that comes with having chronic pain and lessen the perception of pain.

## Different Types of Meditation:

Various meditation methods provide unique ways to shift attention from pain, improve mental clarity, and promote relaxation.

**1.Meditation for Concentration:**
To help focus and minimize distractions, this technique entails focusing on a single point of focus, such as the breath or a mantra. The influence of pain-related thoughts and feelings can be reduced by shifting one's attention.

**2.Metta's Loving-Kindness Meditation:**
Metta meditation encourages kindness and compassion for both oneself and other people. Negative emotional states that are frequently connected to chronic pain can be countered by cultivating positive emotions through Metta.

**3.Body-Scan Meditation:**
This technique entails methodically scanning the body while objectively observing sensations. This technique facilitates

relaxation, helps locate tense spots, and lessens the perceived level of pain.

# Incorporating Yoga for Pain Relief

Yoga combines breathing exercises, meditation, and physical postures to enhance both mental and physical health. Yoga emphasizes gentle movements, breath awareness, and relaxation techniques when customized for people with chronic pain.

## The Effect of Yoga on Pain Management:

Yoga treatments address the mental, emotional, and physical aspects of chronic pain in a comprehensive manner.

**1.Soft Yoga Positions:**
Adapted positions and soft motions emphasize flexibility, strength, and relaxation while taking into account each person's unique capabilities. The goals of these positions are to release tension, lessen stiffness, and enhance general physical function.

**2.Pranayama Breathing Techniques:**
A key component of yoga practice is pranayama, which involves controlled breathing exercises. Methods such as diaphragmatic breathing and alternate nostril breathing help people relax, cope with stress, and manage their perception of pain.

**3.Yoga Nidra:**
 Yoga Nidra, sometimes referred to as "yogic sleep," promotes profound relaxation while preserving consciousness. This technique eases tension brought on by chronic pain, lowers stress levels, and promotes deep relaxation.

# Breathing Exercises

As a means of reducing stress, encouraging relaxation, and assisting with pain modulation, breathing exercises are an essential component of pain management.

## Utilizing the Breath's Power:

Easy methods of pain management, relaxation, and lessening the negative effects of stress on the body include breathing exercises.

**1.Diaphragmatic breathing, also known as deep belly breathing:**
Full contraction of the diaphragm, abdominal expansion, and deep breathing are all part of diaphragmatic breathing. By releasing tense muscles and inducing the body's relaxation response, this technique helps people relax.

**2.Box Breathing Technique:**
 Box breathing calms the nervous system and eases tension, relieving discomfort brought on by pain by having the practitioner inhale, hold, exhale, and hold the breath in equal counts.

**3.Nadi Shodhana (Alternate Nostril Breathing):**
 This pranayama practice alternates between breathing through each nostril. This technique helps reduce stress and pain by balancing energy channels, calming the mind, and encouraging relaxation.

People can take an active role in their pain management journey by incorporating these pain management techniques into their daily routines. People can improve their overall well-being, lessen pain-related distress, and improve their quality of life by practicing yoga, breathing exercises, mindfulness, and attention redirection.

# Chapter 7

# Exercise Strategies for Chronic Pain

A key component of the all-encompassing management of chronic pain is exercise. Personalized exercise regimens, in contrast to popular belief, can significantly improve function, lessen the severity of pain, and improve overall quality of life for people with chronic pain conditions. In the context of managing chronic pain, this chapter examines the value of customized exercise regimens, the function of low-impact and adaptable activities, the significance of consistency, and workable solutions for overcoming exercise barriers.

## Tailored Exercise Plans

### Recognizing Customization

Creating exercise regimens that are specific to each person's needs and abilities is essential for managing chronic pain. These plans create a structured yet flexible approach by taking into account the individual pain condition, general health, fitness level, and any limitations.

### Evaluation and Counseling:

A comprehensive evaluation by a medical specialist, such as a physiotherapist or rehabilitation specialist, is necessary before developing an exercise program. This entails assessing the person's physical state at the moment, determining particular pain triggers, and comprehending any musculoskeletal conditions that may have existed in the past.

## Achieving Practical Objectives:

Customized fitness regimens include goal-setting that is both reasonable and doable. These objectives could be anything from strengthening muscles and tendons to progressively building endurance. People with chronic pain are more motivated and feel like they have accomplished something when they have realistic goals.

## Incorporating Variety:

Variety in exercises prevents monotony and reduces the risk of overuse injuries. Tailored plans may include a combination of aerobic exercises, strength training, flexibility exercises, and functional movements, depending on the individual's preferences and capabilities.

# Adaptive and Low-Impact Activities

## Preserving Mutual Health:

Low-impact and adaptable exercises are essential parts of chronic pain management programs. By minimizing joint stress and lowering the chance of aggravating pain, these exercises lay the groundwork for long-term physical well-being.

## Aquatic and Swimming Exercises:

Because water is buoyant, it has a lessening effect on joints, which makes swimming and other aquatic exercises especially advantageous for people with chronic pain. These exercises strengthen muscles, increase cardiovascular fitness, and create a comfortable atmosphere for movement.

## Cycling and Stationary Biking:

Cycling is a low-impact exercise that improves cardiovascular health and joint mobility. It can be done outside or on a stationary bike. People with different levels of fitness can customize the intensity by varying the resistance.
**Pilates and Yoga:** Core strength, flexibility, and controlled movements are key components of both Pilates and yoga. These practices encourage body awareness and general physical well-being by providing modified poses and exercises appropriate for people with chronic pain.

## Nordic Walking and Walking:

Walking is an easy-to-do, low-impact exercise that works well. With its use of poles, Nordic walking strengthens upper body muscles and improves stability, making it a flexible choice for people who experience chronic pain, especially in the lower limbs.

# Importance of Consistency

## Forming Routines for Extended Advantages:

Achieving the benefits of exercise for managing chronic pain requires consistency. The establishment of a consistent exercise regimen is associated with enhancements in pain thresholds, general physical health, and mental wellness.

## Gradual Progression:

Maintaining consistency entails progressively upping the amount of time, effort, or frequency spent exercising. It is possible to avoid overexertion, lower the risk of injury, and enable the body to adjust to increased activity by gradually increasing from manageable starting levels.
**Monitoring Development:** Recording exercise regimens, pain thresholds, and progress offers important insights. Progress tracking encourages people to keep going, even in the face of small setbacks, and it helps them maintain a positive outlook.

## Including Exercise in Everyday Activities:

Formal sessions are not always necessary for consistent exercise. Including physical activity in everyday activities, like going for quick walks, using the stairs, or stretching during breaks, helps maintain overall consistency and aids in the management of pain.

## Doable Techniques for Application:

Even with an awareness of the advantages of physical activity, people with chronic pain frequently face obstacles that prevent them from participating. Identifying obstacles and putting workable solutions into practice are necessary to get past these barriers.

## Tackling Pain-Related Fear

The fear of making pain worse can be a major obstacle. This is a legitimate fear, and the way to overcome it is to begin with mild exercises and work your way up. Having open lines of communication about concerns with medical professionals guarantees a team approach to pain management.

### Changing Workout Routines:

It is imperative to adjust the exercise regimen if specific exercises are causing pain on a regular basis. This could be switching up the exercises, varying the level of difficulty, or concentrating on distinct muscle groups all while pursuing the overall fitness objective.

### Incorporating Social Support:

Social support can be obtained through working out with a friend, enrolling in group fitness classes, or consulting a fitness expert. Exercise can be more enjoyable and motivating when it is accompanied by encouragement from others and shared experiences.

### Setting Self-Care as a Priority:

Fatigue and erratic energy levels frequently coexist with chronic pain conditions. Setting self-care as a top priority guarantees that the body gets the rest, nutrition, and hydration it needs to prepare for and recover from workouts.

## Including Exercise in Everyday Activities

### Establishing Durable Routines:

A comprehensive strategy that takes into account lifestyle choices, personal preferences, and general well-being is needed to incorporate exercise into daily life. Making exercise a regular part of one's schedule helps people develop long-lasting habits.

## Including Functional Activities:

Functional exercises are applicable and practical because they imitate everyday activities. Regular engagement is ensured by incorporating these exercises into everyday activities, such as squatting to pick up objects or performing seated leg lifts while watching TV.

## Selecting Pleasurable Activities:

Choosing enjoyable activities improves motivation. Exercise can be made enjoyable as a part of daily life by selecting enjoyable activities, such as dancing, gardening, or tai chi.

## Achieving Reasonable Time Commitments:

Exercise is still feasible as long as realistic goals are set and time constraints are acknowledged. Exercise that is focused and short, fitting into daily schedules, is more sustainable than longer irregular sessions.

# Chapter 8

# Nutritional Approaches to Alleviate Pain

A major factor in the management of chronic pain is nutrition. The application of an anti-inflammatory diet, the function of nutritional supplements, and the effect of hydration on pain perception are just a few of the nutritional strategies for pain relief that are covered in this chapter.

## Anti-Inflammatory Diet

### Recognizing the Foundation:

The goal of an anti-inflammatory diet is to lessen the body's internal inflammation, which can affect how pain is perceived. This dietary strategy reduces inflammatory triggers while emphasizing whole, nutrient-dense foods.

### The Significance of Whole Foods:

Whole, unprocessed foods like fruits, vegetables, whole grains, nuts, seeds, and healthy fats like those in fatty fish or olive oil are the mainstays of an anti-inflammatory diet. Antioxidants and phytonutrients found in these foods help to reduce inflammation.

## Fatty Acids Omega-3:

Foods high in omega-3 fatty acids, like walnuts, flaxseeds, and salmon, have strong anti-inflammatory qualities. By balancing the body's inflammatory response, these fatty acids may help lower pain thresholds.

## Reducing Inflammatory Triggers:

Minimizing or eliminating processed foods, sugars, refined carbohydrates, and trans fats is crucial. These items can trigger inflammatory responses in the body, exacerbating pain and discomfort.

# Nutritional Supplements

## Supplementing Your Diet to Enhance It:

Supplements can provide extra help by supplying nutrients that a diet may be deficient in or by having particular anti-inflammatory qualities.

## Omega-3 Supplements:

Concentrated amounts of these vital fatty acids are provided by omega-3 supplements, which include fish oil capsules. Supplements can help reduce inflammation and pain intensity when dietary sources are limited.

## Turmeric, or curcumin:

Turmeric contains a compound called curcumin, which has strong anti-inflammatory effects. Reducing inflammation and pain can be achieved by taking curcumin supplements or adding turmeric to food.

## Vitamin D:

Increased pain perception has been connected to vitamin D deficiency. Taking supplements of vitamin D, particularly for those who are deficient, may aid in the treatment of chronic pain disorders.

# Hydration and Its Impact

## Identifying the Significance:

Maintaining adequate hydration is essential for good health and has a big impact on how people perceive and deal with pain.

## Water for the Health of Tissue:

Sufficient hydration promotes tissue health by lubricating joints and making it easier for nutrients to reach cells. Maintaining adequate hydration is beneficial for better joint function and decreased movement-related pain.

## Minimizing Pain Associated with Dehydration:

Dehydration can make pain that already exists worse by making it more uncomfortable and rigid. Sustaining ideal levels of hydration aid in mitigating these discomforts.

## The Function of Hydration in Overall Health:

Water is essential for good health because it supports many body processes. Adequate hydration promotes detoxification, sharpens the mind, and elevates general health, all of which have a knock-on effect on pain perception.

# Including Nutritional Methods

## Customizing Dietary Practices for Pain Management:

A comprehensive strategy that prioritizes sustainability and balance is needed to incorporate these nutritional approaches into day-to-day living.

## Correcting Macronutrient Balance

Maintaining a healthy balance of proteins, carbs, and healthy fats is important for overall wellbeing. A balanced diet that includes whole grains, lean proteins, and healthy fats helps to manage pain and reduce inflammation.

## Conscientious Consumption:

A positive relationship with food is promoted by mindful eating techniques like savoring meals and being aware of hunger cues. Eating with awareness improves nutrient absorption and digestion, which helps with pain management.

## Steep Adjustments for Sustainability:

Long-term sustainability is ensured by gradually implementing dietary changes. People can make long-lasting dietary improvements and adjust to new eating patterns with gradual modifications.

# A Joint Perspective on Nutrition

## Looking for Expert Advice:

When creating individualized nutritional plans for managing chronic pain, working with healthcare professionals like nutritionists or registered dietitians is essential.

## Personalized Advice:

Experts are able to provide tailored advice based on each person's unique pain condition, food preferences, and overall health. This tailored approach guarantees that dietary modifications are in line with individual needs and objectives.

## Monitoring and Adjusting:

Nutritional plans must be periodically adjusted in addition to being continuously monitored. Health care providers are able to monitor development, make adjustments as needed, and offer continuous assistance, guaranteeing the best possible results with pain management.

# Chapter 9

# Sleep and Its Impact on Chronic Pain

Quality sleep is a critical component of overall well-being, and its relationship with chronic pain is intricate. This chapter delves into the nexus between sleep and chronic pain, exploring sleep disorders associated with persistent pain conditions, the importance of adopting proper sleep hygiene practices, and creating a restful sleep environment to alleviate the challenges posed by chronic pain.

## Sleep Disorders Associated with Chronic Pain

### Comprehending the Interaction:

Sleep and chronic pain have a reciprocal relationship in which each influences the other. Sleep patterns can be disturbed by chronic pain, and vice versa—poor sleep can make pain feel worse.

People who have chronic pain frequently suffer from insomnia, which is characterized by trouble falling or staying asleep. This population may be susceptible to insomnia due to increased sensitivity to stimuli, discomfort during sleep, or anticipation of pain.

### Apnea in Sleep:

Apnea is linked to a higher risk of certain chronic pain conditions, like fibromyalgia. Breathing problems when sleeping not only cause sleep disturbances but also make pain more intense.

### The Syndrome of Restless Legs (RLS):

Those who experience chronic pain frequently report having RLS, which is characterized by an insatiable urge to move the legs. The start and duration of sleep can be hampered by the discomfort brought on by RLS.

### Disorder of Periodic Limb Movement (PLMD):

With PLMD, leg movements are repeated while you sleep, which may wake you up and lead to fragmented sleep. Chronic pain conditions frequently coexist with this disorder.

## Sleep Hygiene Practices

### Developing Restful Sleep Routines:

It's critical for people managing chronic pain to adopt good sleep hygiene practices. The goal of these practices is to maximize the environment that promotes sound sleep.

## Reliable Sleep Pattern:

Even on weekends, keeping a regular sleep schedule entails going to bed and waking up at the same times each day. Maintaining consistency improves the quality of sleep by supporting the body's internal clock.

## Establishing a Calm Sleep Schedule:

Before going to bed, the body receives a signal to wind down from engaging in relaxing activities like reading, light stretching, or mindfulness. Creating a soothing schedule can facilitate falling asleep.

## Reducing Stimulants:

It's critical to stay away from stimulants like caffeine and nicotine right before bed. These drugs may impede one's ability to fall asleep and exacerbate existing sleep disorders.

## Improving the Sleep Environment:

A comfortable mattress and pillows, as well as the control of light and noise levels, all contribute to the creation of a sleep environment that is both comfortable and conducive. These modifications improve the quality of sleep in general.

# Creating a Restful Sleep Environment

## Making the Room Sleep-Friendly:

The physical surroundings in which one sleeps has a big influence on how well they sleep. Addressing a variety of comfort and relaxation-promoting elements is necessary to create a sleep environment that is peaceful and relaxing.

## Achieving the Ideal Room Temperature:

Keeping your room cool and cozy encourages deep, peaceful sleep. Although everyone has a different ideal temperature, it usually ranges from 60 to 67 degrees Fahrenheit (15 to 20 degrees Celsius).

## Managing Light Exposure:

The body's internal clock is regulated when it is exposed to natural light during the day and as little artificial light as possible at night. A good sleeping environment can be produced by using blackout curtains and lowering the lights in the evening.

## Purchasing Comfortable Pillows and Mattress:

Selecting a mattress and pillows is a personal decision that depends on personal tastes and any musculoskeletal disorders that may already be present. To encourage restorative sleep, it is essential to spend money on pillows and mattresses that offer adequate comfort and support.

## Minimizing Disturbances and Noise:

Soundproofing techniques, white noise generators, and earplugs can all help reduce noise disturbances. The ability to fall asleep and stay asleep is improved by creating a quiet sleeping environment.

# Including Techniques to Get Better Sleep

## Holistic Methods for Treating Pain and Sleep:

A comprehensive strategy that takes into account all the variables influencing chronic pain management and the quality of sleep is needed to incorporate sleep techniques into everyday activities.

## Physical Mind-Body Methods:

Techniques like mindfulness meditation, progressive muscle relaxation, and guided imagery can help you relax and go to sleep more easily. These methods have a beneficial effect on chronic pain by reducing stress overall as well.

## Physical Activity:

Regular exercise that is catered to each person's abilities promotes better sleep. Exercise improves mood, lowers anxiety, and improves general wellbeing, all of which have a beneficial effect on the quality of sleep.

## Cognitive Behavioral Therapy for Insomnia (CBT-I):

CBT-I is an evidence-based therapeutic approach specifically designed to address insomnia. It involves identifying and changing negative thought patterns and behaviors that contribute to sleep difficulties.

## Medication Management:

In some cases, healthcare providers may recommend medications to address sleep disturbances. These may include sleep aids or medications targeting underlying pain conditions that impact sleep.

# Looking for Professional Advice

## Working Together for the Best Results:

Getting expert advice is essential for people navigating these difficulties because of the complex relationship between chronic pain and sleep.

## Advisory Sleep Consultants:

To identify particular sleep disorders and customize interventions, sleep specialists can perform comprehensive assessments. In order to assess sleep patterns and disturbances more thoroughly, diagnostic sleep studies might be advised.

## Working Together with Pain Management Experts:

A comprehensive approach to treating both pain and sleep is ensured through collaborative efforts between pain management professionals and sleep specialists. Getting the best results is more likely when care is coordinated.

## Personalized Care Plans:

To address both sleep and chronic pain, professionals can create customized treatment plans that may involve a mix of targeted approaches, medications, and behavioral interventions.

# Chapter 10

# Mind-Body Therapies and Their Role

Mind-body therapies encompass a spectrum of approaches that emphasize the connection between mental, emotional, and physical health. In the context of chronic pain management, these therapies offer valuable tools to alleviate pain, reduce stress, and improve overall well-being. This chapter delves into the role and benefits of cognitive-behavioral therapy (CBT), biofeedback, guided imagery, music therapy, and art therapy in addressing chronic pain.

## Cognitive Behavioral Therapy (CBT)

### Restructuring Thoughts and Behaviors:

CBT is a therapeutic approach that focuses on altering negative thought patterns and behaviors contributing to emotional distress and physical symptoms, including pain.

### Changing Thought Patterns:

CBT helps individuals identify and challenge negative thought patterns associated with pain. By reframing thoughts from catastrophizing to more adaptive ones, individuals can reduce the emotional impact of pain.

## Behavioral Techniques:

CBT incorporates behavioral strategies to manage pain, such as activity pacing, relaxation techniques, and gradual exposure to activities that may evoke pain. These techniques help individuals regain a sense of control over their pain experience.

## Addressing Emotional Components:

By addressing underlying emotional components linked to pain, such as anxiety or depression, CBT contributes to improved pain management and enhances coping mechanisms.

# Biofeedback

## Harnessing Body Signals for Control:

Biofeedback is a technique that enables individuals to gain awareness and voluntary control over physiological processes like heart rate, muscle tension, and skin temperature, often related to pain experiences.

## Promoting self-regulation:

Biofeedback devices provide real-time feedback about bodily functions, allowing individuals to learn how to modify these functions consciously. Through practice, individuals can gain control over physiological responses associated with pain.

## Muscle Relaxation:

Biofeedback often incorporates techniques for relaxation, such as progressive muscle relaxation or diaphragmatic breathing. These practices aid in reducing muscle tension and alleviating pain-related symptoms.

## Enhancing Mind-Body Connection:

Biofeedback fosters awareness of the mind-body connection, empowering individuals to recognize and modify physical responses to stressors or pain triggers.

# Guided Image

## Harnessing the Power of Visualization:

Guided imagery involves using mental images to evoke relaxation responses, redirect attention away from pain, and promote a sense of calmness.

## Creating Mental Pictures:

Guided imagery sessions involve visualizing peaceful and serene scenes, such as a tranquil beach or a serene forest. This mental imagery facilitates relaxation and distracts from pain sensations.

## Reducing Stress Responses:

Engaging in guided imagery exercises decreases stress hormones, promoting relaxation and reducing the physiological arousal associated with pain.

Guided imagery empowers individuals to develop coping strategies, fostering a sense of control over their pain experiences and improving overall well-being.

# Music and Art Therapy

## Creative Approaches to Healing:

Music and art therapies leverage creative expressions to address emotional, psychological, and physical aspects of chronic pain.

## Music Therapy:

Engaging with music, whether listening, playing instruments, or singing, has therapeutic effects on pain management. Music reduces anxiety, improves mood, and distracts individuals from pain sensations.

## Art Therapy:

Expressive activities like drawing, painting, or sculpting provide avenues for emotional expression and stress relief. Art therapy encourages individuals to explore and process emotions related to their pain experiences.

## Promoting Relaxation and Distraction:

Both music and art therapies offer avenues for relaxation and distraction, diverting attention away from pain while providing avenues for emotional release and creativity.

# Integrating Mind-Body Therapies

## Holistic Approaches to Pain Management:

Integrating mind-body therapies into pain management strategies involves considering individual preferences, needs, and the holistic nature of healing.

## Combining Therapies:

Integrating multiple mind-body therapies allows individuals to access a range of techniques, addressing different aspects of pain and emotional distress. Combining CBT with biofeedback or guided imagery, for instance, offers a comprehensive approach.

## Tailoring to Individual Needs:

Recognizing that not all mind-body therapies work universally for everyone, tailoring approaches to individual preferences and responses ensures greater efficacy.

## Collaborative Efforts:

Collaborating with healthcare providers and therapists ensures a coordinated approach to pain management, incorporating mind-body therapies alongside other treatments.

# Professional Guidance and Support

## Navigating Mind-Body Therapies:

Seeking guidance from trained professionals specializing in mind-body therapies ensures safe and effective implementation.

### Qualified Practitioners:

Working with licensed therapists or healthcare providers trained in mind-body therapies ensures appropriate guidance and support tailored to individual needs.

### Personalized Plans:

Professionals develop personalized plans, incorporating specific mind-body techniques that align with an individual's goals and pain management needs.

### Evaluating Progress:

Regular evaluation and monitoring of progress help adjust mind-body therapy approaches as needed, ensuring optimal outcomes in chronic pain management.

# Chapter 11

# Complementary Therapies

Complementary therapies offer diverse modalities that complement traditional medical approaches in addressing chronic pain. This chapter explores several effective complementary therapies, including Acupuncture and Acupressure, Chiropractic Care, Herbal Remedies, and Massage Therapy, shedding light on their applications and benefits in managing chronic pain conditions.

## Acupuncture and Acupressure

### Stimulating Vital Energy Points:

Acupuncture and acupressure are rooted in Traditional Chinese Medicine (TCM) and focus on stimulating specific points on the body to restore the flow of vital energy, known as Qi, and alleviate pain.

### Acupuncture:

In acupuncture, fine needles are inserted into specific points along meridians believed to correspond with different organs and body functions. This stimulation is thought to rebalance energy flow and reduce pain perception.

### Acupressure:

Acupressure involves applying pressure to the same points used in acupuncture, but without the use of needles. Pressure is applied using fingers, palms, or devices, aiming to achieve similar pain relief benefits as acupuncture.

## Pain Management Effects:

Both acupuncture and acupressure are known for their potential to relieve various types of chronic pain, including musculoskeletal pain, headaches, and neuropathic pain, by promoting the release of endorphins and modulating pain signals.

# Chiropractic Care

## Aligning Spinal Health:

Chiropractic care focuses on diagnosing and treating musculoskeletal disorders, primarily through manual adjustments to the spine and other joints.

## Spinal Manipulation:

Chiropractors use hands-on spinal manipulation techniques to realign the musculoskeletal structure, aiming to improve spinal function and alleviate pain caused by misalignments or imbalances.

## Pain Alleviation:

Chiropractic care is commonly sought for managing back pain, neck pain, and joint-related discomfort. The adjustments aim to relieve pressure on affected nerves and restore normal joint movement, potentially reducing pain.

## Holistic Approach:

Chiropractors often take a holistic approach, considering lifestyle modifications, exercises, and ergonomic recommendations to complement spinal adjustments and enhance overall musculoskeletal health.

# Herbal Remedies

## Natural Approaches to Pain Relief:

Herbal remedies encompass a wide array of plant-based preparations and supplements used to alleviate pain and inflammation, drawing from various traditional healing practices.

## Natural Anti-inflammatories:

Certain herbs, such as turmeric (containing curcumin), ginger, and boswellia, possess anti-inflammatory properties that may help reduce pain associated with inflammation in conditions like arthritis.

## Analgesic Effects:

Herbal remedies like Devil's Claw, White Willow Bark (source of salicin, akin to aspirin), and Arnica are believed to have analgesic effects, potentially reducing pain intensity when used appropriately.

## Caution and Consultation:

While herbal remedies offer natural alternatives, it's crucial to use them judiciously and consult healthcare professionals due to potential interactions with medications and varying levels of scientific evidence supporting their efficacy.

## Massage Therapy

### Therapeutic Touch for Pain Relief:

Massage therapy involves manipulating soft tissues, muscles, and connective tissues through various techniques to promote relaxation, alleviate muscle tension, and reduce pain.

### Types of Massage:

Techniques such as Swedish massage, deep tissue massage, myofascial release, and trigger point therapy are commonly used in managing chronic pain conditions.

### Pain Reduction Mechanisms:

Massage therapy improves circulation, relaxes muscles, and stimulates the release of endorphins and serotonin. These effects contribute to pain reduction, easing tension, and promoting a sense of well-being.

### Integration into pain management plans :

Massage therapy is often integrated into comprehensive pain management plans, offering not only physical benefits but also psychological relief and stress reduction.

# Integrating Complementary Therapies in Pain Management

## Collaborative and Personalized Approaches:

The  integration of complementary therapies in chronic pain management involves collaboration between patients, healthcare providers, and practitioners of these modalities.

## Comprehensive Treatment Plans:

Complementary therapies are often integrated into comprehensive pain management plans, incorporating various modalities to address the multifaceted aspects of chronic pain.

## Personalized Approaches:

Tailoring complementary therapies to individual needs and preferences ensures optimal outcomes. This individualization accounts for the specific pain condition, medical history, and responsiveness to different modalities.

## Combining Therapies:

Integrating multiple complementary therapies or combining them with conventional treatments, when appropriate, may yield synergistic effects, enhancing overall pain relief and functional improvement.

# Chapter 12

# Dealing with Stigma and Social Judgment

The stigma surrounding chronic pain poses significant challenges for individuals managing these conditions. This chapter delves into strategies for addressing stigma, raising awareness, advocating for chronic pain recognition, and dispelling misconceptions to foster greater understanding and support.

## Understanding Stigma in Chronic Pain

### The Burden of Misunderstanding:

Chronic pain, often an invisible condition, faces misconceptions and societal biases, leading to stigma. The lack of visible symptoms or definitive diagnostic tests often results in skepticism, disbelief, or dismissiveness from others.

### Invisibility of Pain:

The subjective nature of chronic pain makes it difficult for others to comprehend its severity or impact. This invisibility leads to skepticism and misconceptions, compounding the challenges faced by individuals with chronic pain.

## Social Isolation and Misjudgment:

Stigma and judgment can lead to social isolation, strained relationships, and feelings of being misunderstood or unsupported. The negative impact on mental health often exacerbates the pain experience.

# Raising Awareness

## Educating to Combat Stigma:

Raising awareness about chronic pain is pivotal in dispelling misconceptions and fostering empathy and understanding among the public.

## Educational Campaigns:

Initiatives aimed at educating the public about chronic pain, its prevalence, and its diverse manifestations play a crucial role. These campaigns aim to sensitize communities, healthcare providers, and policymakers to the challenges faced by individuals with chronic pain.

## Sharing Personal Stories:

Personal narratives from individuals living with chronic pain humanize the experience and provide insight into the daily struggles faced. Sharing stories of resilience and courage can help dispel myths and encourage empathy.

## Community Engagement:

Engaging local communities through workshops, seminars, or support groups fosters understanding and empathy. These platforms offer spaces for discussions, knowledge sharing, and mutual support.

# Advocacy for Chronic Pain Recognition

## Fostering Systemic Change:

Advocacy efforts play a vital role in advancing policies and practices that recognize chronic pain as a legitimate health issue deserving of support and understanding.

## Policy Initiatives:

Advocacy groups and organizations work towards influencing policy changes that prioritize chronic pain management, ensuring access to adequate healthcare, pain management resources, and disability support.

## Healthcare Provider Education:

Training healthcare professionals to better understand and address chronic pain reduces the likelihood of dismissiveness and ensures patients receive compassionate and effective care.

## Legitimizing Patient Experiences:

Advocacy efforts aim to legitimize the experiences of individuals with chronic pain, ensuring their voices are heard in shaping healthcare policies, research funding, and societal attitudes.

# Addressing Misconceptions

## Challenging Preconceived Notions:

Addressing and dispelling misconceptions surrounding chronic pain is crucial for fostering empathy and support from society at large.

## Myth-Busting Efforts:

Debunking myths and misconceptions through factual information and evidence-based research is essential. Correcting false beliefs about chronic pain contributes to a more supportive environment.

## Highlighting the Multifaceted Nature of Pain:

Educating others about the complex nature of chronic pain, its varied manifestations, and its impact on physical, emotional, and social well-being helps combat oversimplified perceptions.

## Empathy and Validation:

Encouraging empathetic responses and validating the experiences of individuals with chronic pain fosters a supportive and understanding environment. Acknowledging the legitimacy of their experiences is crucial in reducing stigma.

# Coping Strategies for Individuals

## Building Resilience in the Face of Stigma:

Empowering individuals with chronic pain with coping strategies to navigate societal judgment and stigma is integral for their mental well-being.

## Self-Advocacy and Communication:

Equipping individuals with tools for effective communication about their pain experience aids in advocating for their needs and fostering understanding among friends, family, and healthcare providers.

## Building a Support Network:

Encouraging individuals to build a support network of understanding friends, family, or support groups provides validation, empathy, and a sense of belonging, countering the effects of social isolation.

## Promoting Self-Care:

Encouraging self-care practices, stress management techniques, and seeking professional support for mental health needs assists individuals in managing the emotional toll of societal judgment and stigma.

# Chapter 13

# Effective Communication with Loved Ones and Healthcare Providers

Communication plays a pivotal role in the journey of managing chronic pain. This chapter explores the nuances of open communication strategies, building a supportive network, and advocating for one's needs within both personal relationships and the healthcare system.

## Open Communication Strategies

### Navigating Dialogue with Clarity:

Effective communication is the cornerstone of building understanding and support. For individuals grappling with chronic pain, expressing their experiences and needs requires thoughtful and open dialogue.

### Expressing Pain Levels and Variability:

Describing the varying levels and nuances of pain helps loved ones and healthcare providers comprehend the dynamic nature of chronic pain. Utilizing pain scales or descriptive language can convey the intensity, frequency, and impact on daily life.

### Articulating Emotional Responses:

Chronic pain often intertwines with emotional struggles. Communicating these emotional responses, whether frustration, sadness, or anxiety, provides insight into the holistic impact of pain on mental well-being.

### Using "I" Statements:

Framing conversations using "I" statements, such as "I feel" or "I need," promotes personal responsibility and avoids placing blame. This approach encourages open dialogue and reduces defensiveness.

### Discussing Treatment Preferences:

Engaging in discussions about treatment preferences, including medication options, therapeutic approaches, and lifestyle modifications, ensures collaborative decision-making and enhances treatment adherence.

## Building a Supportive Network

### Fostering Understanding and Empathy:

Chronic pain can strain personal relationships, making it essential to cultivate a supportive network that understands and empathizes with the challenges faced.

### Educating Loved Ones:

Providing educational resources or inviting loved ones to participate in support groups or counseling sessions fosters understanding. Educated support networks are better equipped to offer empathy and encouragement.

## Setting Realistic Expectations:

Communicating limitations and setting realistic expectations help manage the potential strain chronic pain can place on relationships. Setting boundaries and finding a balance between independence and needed assistance is crucial.

## Encouraging Open Dialogue:

Creating an environment where open communication is welcomed encourages loved ones to express their concerns, ask questions, and provide support without judgment. Transparency strengthens the bond between individuals and their support network.

## Sharing Coping Strategies:

Introducing loved ones to effective coping strategies, whether attending doctor's appointments together, practicing relaxation techniques, or participating in enjoyable activities, encourages a shared understanding of how to navigate the challenges of chronic pain collectively.

# Advocating for Your Needs

## Empowering Individuals in Healthcare Settings:

Effective communication extends beyond personal relationships to interactions within the healthcare system. Advocating for one's needs is essential for receiving comprehensive and patient-centered care.

## Preparing for Medical Appointments:

 Prior to medical appointments, individuals can prepare by documenting symptoms, tracking pain patterns, and noting questions or concerns. This preparation ensures a more focused and productive conversation with healthcare providers.

## Clearly Expressing Symptoms:

 Articulating symptoms with precision, including the location, duration, and impact on daily life, aids healthcare providers in accurate diagnosis and treatment planning. Clear communication facilitates a more collaborative approach to care.

## Discussing Treatment Preferences:

 In addition to personal preferences, discussing treatment goals, potential side effects, and desired outcomes ensures that healthcare providers align treatment plans with the individual's values and priorities.

## Seeking Clarification and Asking Questions:

Actively engaging in conversations with healthcare providers involves seeking clarification about medical terminology, asking questions about treatment options, and expressing any concerns. This approach fosters a sense of partnership in the decision-making process.

# Overcoming Challenges in Communication

## Strategies for Resilience:

Despite the importance of effective communication, challenges may arise. Addressing these challenges requires resilience and adaptability.

## Managing Frustration and Misunderstanding:

Chronic pain can lead to frustration, and misunderstandings may occur. Developing patience and finding alternative ways to express oneself during challenging moments can help navigate these situations.

## Seeking mediation or counselling:

In instances where communication breakdowns persist, seeking the assistance of a mediator or counselor can provide guidance. Professional support offers strategies for improving communication within personal relationships.

## Building a Collaborative Relationship with Healthcare Providers:

Collaborating with healthcare providers involves establishing a partnership built on trust and mutual respect. If challenges arise, expressing concerns and working together to find solutions strengthens the therapeutic alliance.

# Chapter 14

# Navigating Finances, Insurance, and Disability.

Managing chronic pain goes beyond medical considerations; it also involves navigating the intricate landscape of finances, insurance coverage, and potential disability. This chapter delves into the essential aspects of understanding insurance, navigating disability processes, and financial planning tailored to the unique challenges posed by chronic pain.

## Understanding Insurance Coverage

### Unraveling the Complexities:

Understanding insurance coverage is a crucial aspect of chronic pain management, ensuring individuals have access to necessary medical treatments and services.

### Reviewing Policy Terms:

Thoroughly reviewing insurance policy terms helps individuals understand coverage limitations, including copayments, deductibles, and out-of-pocket expenses. Awareness of policy specifics empowers individuals to make informed decisions about their healthcare.

## Inquiring about Pain Management Services:

Insurance policies vary in coverage for pain management services. Inquiring about coverage for physical therapy, medications, and alternative therapies such as acupuncture or chiropractic care ensures individuals explore available options within their coverage.

## Confirming Prescription Medication Coverage:

Chronic pain often involves medications. Confirming coverage for prescription medications, including generic and brand-name options, aids in financial planning and avoids unexpected costs.

## Exploring Mental Health Coverage:

Chronic pain is closely linked to mental health. Understanding coverage for mental health services, counseling, and therapy ensures comprehensive support for the emotional aspects of chronic pain.

# Navigating Disability Processes

## Advocating for Support:

For individuals whose chronic pain significantly impacts their ability to work, navigating disability processes becomes a crucial aspect of financial stability and support.

## Understanding Eligibility Criteria:

Familiarizing oneself with eligibility criteria for disability benefits is the first step. Criteria often consider the severity of the condition, its impact on daily functioning, and the ability to engage in gainful employment.

## Medical Documentation:

Compiling thorough medical documentation is essential. This includes medical records, diagnoses, treatment plans, and statements from healthcare providers detailing the impact of chronic pain on daily activities and work capacity.

## Engaging Healthcare Providers:

Collaborating with healthcare providers is integral. Requesting their support in providing comprehensive and detailed documentation strengthens the disability application, offering a more accurate representation of the individual's condition.

## Seeking Legal Guidance if Necessary:

Disability processes can be complex, and denials are not uncommon. In cases of denials, seeking legal guidance from disability attorneys with expertise in navigating appeals processes can be invaluable.

# Financial Planning for Chronic Pain

## Tailoring Strategies to Individual Needs:

Chronic pain often introduces financial challenges, from medical expenses to potential changes in employment status. Strategic financial planning helps individuals proactively address these challenges.

## Budgeting for Medical Expenses:

Creating a budget that accounts for medical expenses, including copayments, prescription costs, and potential out-of-pocket expenditures for treatments, ensures financial preparedness for healthcare-related costs.

## Emergency Fund Planning:

Establishing an emergency fund becomes crucial for unforeseen circumstances. Chronic pain may lead to unexpected flare-ups or changes in employment, making an emergency fund a valuable resource during challenging times.

## Exploring Disability Insurance Options:

Individuals employed or seeking employment should explore disability insurance options. Disability insurance provides financial protection in the event chronic pain leads to the inability to work, offering income replacement during disability.

## Consulting Financial Advisors:

Seeking guidance from financial advisors helps individuals tailor financial plans to their unique circumstances. Advisors can offer insights into investment strategies, retirement planning, and navigating changes in income due to chronic pain.

# Overcoming Financial Challenges

## Strategies for Resilience:

Navigating the financial aspects of chronic pain requires resilience and adaptability. Strategies to overcome financial challenges contribute to long-term stability.

### Negotiating Medical Bills:

When faced with high medical bills, negotiating with healthcare providers or facilities can lead to reduced costs or structured payment plans. Many providers are willing to work with individuals facing financial constraints.

### Exploring Assistance Programs:

Investigating available assistance programs, both at the local and national levels, can provide additional support. Some programs offer financial assistance, discounted medications, or subsidized healthcare services.

### Seeking Employment Accommodations:

For individuals employed while managing chronic pain, exploring workplace accommodations can be beneficial. This may involve flexible work hours, ergonomic adjustments, or remote work options, contributing to sustained employment.

### Staying Informed about Policy Changes:

Staying informed about changes in healthcare policies, disability regulations, or financial assistance programs ensures individuals are aware of potential benefits or adjustments that may alleviate financial burdens.

# Chapter 15

# Managing Stress and Emotions

Chronic pain extends beyond physical discomfort; it intricately intertwines with emotional well-being, often posing significant challenges. This chapter delves into the multifaceted aspects of managing stress and emotions associated with chronic pain, emphasizing the recognition of emotional impact, stress management techniques, and the importance of seeking professional support.

## Recognizing Emotional Impact

### Unveiling the Complex Connection:

Chronic pain and emotions are intricately linked, creating a dynamic interplay that can significantly impact an individual's mental well-being.

### Pain and Emotional Centers:

Chronic pain activates brain regions associated with emotions. The prolonged sensory input from pain signals can lead to changes in emotional processing, potentially resulting in heightened stress, anxiety, depression, or mood fluctuations.

### Impact on Quality of Life:

Emotional responses to chronic pain can profoundly affect an individual's quality of life. Persistent pain may contribute to feelings of frustration, helplessness, isolation, and a sense of loss

as individuals navigate changes in daily activities and
relationships.

## Cyclical Nature:

 Emotional distress can, in turn, influence the perception and
intensity of pain. Stress and negative emotions may exacerbate
pain, creating a cyclical relationship where pain and emotions
reinforce each other.

## Communication Challenges:

 Expressing emotional distress related to chronic pain can be
challenging. Societal expectations, fear of judgment, or the desire
to maintain a stoic façade may hinder open communication about
the emotional impact of pain.

# Stress Management Techniques

## Empowering Strategies for Coping:

Effective stress management techniques play a crucial role in
mitigating the emotional toll of chronic pain, fostering resilience,
and improving overall well-being.

## Mindfulness and Meditation:

Mindfulness practices, including meditation, cultivate awareness
of the present moment. These techniques help individuals detach
from distressing thoughts, reduce anxiety, and enhance overall
emotional resilience.

## Deep Breathing Exercises:

Incorporating deep breathing exercises promotes relaxation and helps manage stress. Techniques such as diaphragmatic breathing or paced breathing can elicit a calming response, easing tension associated with chronic pain.

## Progressive Muscle Relaxation (PMR):

PMR involves systematically tensing and relaxing muscle groups, promoting physical and mental relaxation. This technique can alleviate muscle tension linked to chronic pain and contribute to stress reduction.

## Cognitive Behavioral Therapy (CBT):

CBT is a therapeutic approach that addresses negative thought patterns and behaviors. In the context of chronic pain, CBT helps individuals reframe thoughts, manage stressors, and develop effective coping strategies.

## Engaging in Relaxation Activities:

Activities such as listening to calming music, engaging in hobbies, or spending time in nature provide avenues for relaxation and emotional relief. Identifying enjoyable and soothing activities contributes to a holistic stress management plan.

# Seeking Professional Support

## The Role of Mental Health Professionals:

Recognizing the complexity of emotional responses to chronic pain, seeking professional support becomes an essential component of comprehensive care.

## Psychologists and Counselors:

Mental health professionals, such as psychologists and counselors, specialize in addressing the emotional impact of chronic pain. They provide a safe space for individuals to explore their feelings, develop coping strategies, and navigate the challenges of living with chronic pain.

## Pain Psychologists:

Pain psychologists specialize in the intersection of pain and psychology. They offer tailored interventions, including cognitive-behavioral therapies, biofeedback, and pain education, to address both the physical and emotional aspects of chronic pain.

## Psychiatric Support:

In cases where chronic pain contributes to severe anxiety or depression, psychiatric support may be beneficial. Psychiatric medications, when prescribed by healthcare professionals, can assist in managing emotional symptoms associated with chronic pain.

## Support Groups and Peer Counseling:

Engaging in support groups or peer counseling allows individuals to connect with others facing similar challenges. Sharing experiences, strategies, and emotional support within a supportive community can be a valuable aspect of emotional well-being.

# Integrating Emotional Management into Daily Life

## Holistic Approaches:

Managing stress and emotions associated with chronic pain is an ongoing process that requires the integration of holistic approaches into daily life.

## Daily Mindfulness Practices:

Incorporating brief mindfulness practices into daily routines, such as mindful breathing or short meditation sessions, fosters emotional resilience. Consistency in these practices contributes to long-term stress management.

## Setting Realistic Goals:

Establishing realistic and achievable goals, both in managing chronic pain and emotional well-being, promotes a sense of accomplishment. Breaking down larger goals into smaller, manageable steps ensures progress and reduces feelings of overwhelm.

## Maintaining Social Connections:

Nurturing social connections, whether through friends, family, or support groups, provides emotional support. Regular interactions with loved ones contribute to a sense of belonging and reduce feelings of isolation.

## Prioritizing Self-Care:

Prioritizing self-care activities, including adequate sleep, balanced nutrition, and regular physical activity, supports overall well-being. These foundational elements contribute to physical and emotional resilience.

# Chapter 16

# Employment Challenges and Coping Strategies

Navigating the intersection of chronic pain and employment presents unique challenges for individuals striving to balance their health needs with professional responsibilities. This chapter explores the complexities of employment challenges in the context of chronic pain, encompassing workplace accommodations, strategies for balancing work and health, and coping mechanisms for those considering or undergoing career changes.

## Workplace Accommodations

### Fostering Inclusive Work Environments:

Workplace accommodations play a crucial role in empowering individuals with chronic pain to maintain gainful employment and contribute effectively to their organizations.

### Open Communication with Employers:

Establishing open communication with employers about chronic pain is essential. Sharing information about the condition, its impact on daily functioning, and potential workplace challenges creates a foundation for collaboration.

### Requesting Reasonable Accommodations:

The Americans with Disabilities Act (ADA) and similar legislations globally emphasize the provision of reasonable accommodations.

These may include adjustments to work schedules, modifications to physical workspaces, or flexible policies related to breaks and attendance.

## Ergonomic Workstations:

Ensuring an ergonomic workstation contributes to pain management. Adjustments such as proper chair support, ergonomic desks, and appropriate lighting can alleviate physical strain and promote comfort.

## Flexible Work Arrangements:

Exploring flexible work arrangements, such as remote work options or adjusted hours, enables individuals to manage chronic pain more effectively while fulfilling work responsibilities.

# Balancing Work and Health

## Strategies for Sustainable Employment:

Balancing the demands of work with the health challenges posed by chronic pain requires intentional strategies to foster a sustainable and supportive professional environment.

## Prioritizing Self-Care during Work Hours:

Incorporating self-care practices within the workday is crucial. Short breaks for stretching or relaxation exercises, maintaining hydration, and adhering to prescribed medication schedules contribute to overall well-being.

## Time Management and Pacing:

Effective time management and pacing strategies help individuals distribute their energy throughout the workday. Prioritizing tasks, breaking down projects into manageable steps, and incorporating regular breaks prevent burnout and reduce the risk of exacerbating pain.

## Building a Supportive Work Culture:

Fostering a supportive work culture involves cultivating empathy and understanding among colleagues and supervisors. Encouraging open communication, raising awareness about chronic pain, and promoting inclusivity contribute to a positive and supportive workplace environment.

## Utilizing Employee Assistance Programs (EAPs):

Many organizations offer Employee Assistance Programs that provide support for mental health and well-being. Accessing EAP services can offer counseling, resources, and strategies for managing stress associated with chronic pain.

# Coping with Career Changes

## Navigating Transitions:

Chronic pain may prompt individuals to consider or undergo career changes. Coping with these transitions involves strategic planning and resilience.

## Assessing Career Goals and Values:

Reflecting on career goals, values, and personal priorities is fundamental when contemplating a career change. Aligning professional pursuits with individual values contributes to greater job satisfaction.

## Exploring Transferable Skills:

Identifying transferable skills gained from previous roles ensures a smooth transition into new career paths. These skills may include communication, problem-solving, project management, and adaptability.

## Networking and Seeking Guidance:

Networking within professional circles and seeking guidance from mentors or career counselors offers valuable insights. Networking can unveil new opportunities, and guidance from experienced professionals aids in informed decision-making.

## Considering Flexible Work Options:

Exploring careers with flexible work options, such as freelance work, consulting, or part-time positions, accommodates the fluctuating nature of chronic pain. Flexibility in work arrangements provides individuals with greater control over their schedules.

## Overcoming Emotional Challenges

## Strategies for Resilience:

The process of managing employment challenges and potential career changes due to chronic pain is not without emotional challenges. Implementing resilience strategies is crucial for maintaining a positive mindset.

## Acceptance and Adaptability:

Acknowledging and accepting the impact of chronic pain on career aspirations is the first step. Embracing adaptability allows individuals to explore alternative paths without feeling constrained by perceived limitations.

## Seeking Emotional Support:

Emotional support from friends, family, or support groups helps individuals cope with the emotional challenges of career changes. Sharing concerns, fears, and aspirations provides a supportive outlet for processing these transitions.

## Professional Mental Health Support:

Engaging with mental health professionals or career counselors during periods of transition offers targeted support. These professionals assist individuals in managing stress, addressing emotional challenges, and developing coping strategies.

## Maintaining a Positive Mindset:

Cultivating a positive mindset involves focusing on strengths, achievements, and opportunities rather than dwelling on challenges. Recognizing personal resilience and the capacity for growth fosters optimism during times of change

# Chapter 17

# Support Networks and Community Resources

Navigating chronic pain often necessitates a robust support network and access to community resources that offer understanding, guidance, and solidarity. This chapter delves into the significance of support groups, online communities, and local resources and organizations as essential components of comprehensive chronic pain management.

## Joining Support Groups

### Fostering Understanding and Connection:

Support groups serve as invaluable platforms for individuals experiencing chronic pain to connect, share experiences, and offer mutual support.

### Shared Experiences and Empathy:

Participating in support groups facilitates interactions with individuals facing similar challenges. Sharing personal experiences fosters empathy, validates feelings, and helps individuals feel understood and less isolated.

## Access to Practical Advice:

Support groups offer a wealth of practical advice and coping strategies derived from collective experiences. Individuals can learn about effective pain management techniques, treatments, and lifestyle adjustments from others who have navigated similar journeys.

## Emotional Support and Encouragement:

Engaging in conversations within support groups provides emotional support and encouragement. Encouraging words, shared victories, and understanding create a sense of camaraderie and motivation.

## Opportunities for Advocacy and Awareness:

Support groups often engage in advocacy efforts to raise awareness about chronic pain conditions. Participating in advocacy initiatives empowers individuals to amplify their voices and drive societal understanding and change.

# Online Communities

## Accessible Platforms for Connection:

Online communities offer accessible spaces for individuals experiencing chronic pain to connect, seek advice, and share resources regardless of geographical limitations.

## 24/7 Accessibility and Global Reach:

Online communities transcend geographical barriers, allowing individuals worldwide to connect at any time. This accessibility ensures continuous support, regardless of time zones or physical location.

## Diverse Perspectives and Information Sharing:

Online platforms bring together individuals from various backgrounds and experiences. This diversity fosters the sharing of a wide array of perspectives, treatment options, and coping mechanisms for chronic pain.

## Anonymity and Privacy:

Some individuals prefer the anonymity provided by online communities. Anonymity allows individuals to share their experiences and concerns openly while maintaining their privacy, which can be comforting for those hesitant to discuss chronic pain in a public setting.

## Access to Expert Advice and Resources:

Many online communities host discussions with healthcare professionals or offer access to reputable resources and articles, empowering members with information and guidance from experts.

# Local Resources and Organizations

## Tapping into Community Support:

Local resources and organizations offer tangible assistance and support tailored to the needs of individuals experiencing chronic pain within their specific communities.

## Access to Local Services:

Local resources often provide access to healthcare professionals specializing in chronic pain management, such as pain clinics, physical therapists, or specialized care centers.

## Supportive Workshops and Events:

Many local organizations host workshops, seminars, or events focused on chronic pain management. These events offer educational opportunities, practical advice, and networking opportunities with other individuals and healthcare professionals.

## Navigating Financial and Legal Aspects:

Local resources assist individuals in navigating financial aspects, insurance queries, or legal challenges related to chronic pain. They offer guidance on available assistance programs and potential avenues for financial support.

## Community Engagement and Advocacy:

Engaging with local organizations promotes community awareness and advocacy efforts related to chronic pain. Participating in local events or campaigns helps raise awareness, reduce stigma, and advocate for better resources and support.

# Integration of Community Resources

## Creating a Holistic Support System:

The integration of support groups, online communities, and local resources and organizations contributes to a holistic and comprehensive approach to managing chronic pain.

## Utilizing Various Channels for Support:

Engaging with multiple support channels ensures a diverse range of support mechanisms. Combining in-person interactions, online engagement, and local resources maximizes access to support and resources.

## Building Long-Term Connections:

Nurturing connections within support groups, online communities, and local organizations fosters long-term relationships. Consistent engagement builds trust and ensures a sustained network of support.

## Encouraging Active Participation:

Encouraging active participation in these communities empowers individuals to contribute their experiences, insights, and support to others navigating similar challenges. Active participation enriches the collective knowledge and support available within these communities.

## Seeking and Offering Support:

Recognizing that seeking support is as crucial as offering support contributes to a reciprocal and supportive community. By both seeking guidance and providing assistance when possible, individuals create a symbiotic network of support.

# Chapter 18

# Research, Innovations, and Future Perspectives

The final chapter of our journey through chronic pain management explores the dynamic landscape of research, technological advancements, and the promising horizons of future treatments. In this chapter, we delve into the current state of research in chronic pain, the transformative impact of technological innovations, and the hope that emerging treatments bring to individuals grappling with persistent pain.

## Current Research in Chronic Pain

### Unveiling Insights and Breakthroughs:

The field of chronic pain research is continuously evolving, driven by a collective commitment to understanding the intricate mechanisms underlying pain and developing more effective interventions.

### Neurobiology and Pain Pathways:

Current research focuses on unraveling the neurobiological intricacies of pain. Scientists explore pain pathways, neurotransmitter interactions, and the role of the central nervous system, aiming to pinpoint targets for novel therapeutic interventions.

## Genetic and Epigenetic Factors:

The exploration of genetic and epigenetic factors contributing to chronic pain is a burgeoning area of research. Identifying genetic predispositions and understanding how environmental factors influence gene expression holds promise for personalized treatment approaches.

## Innovations in Imaging Technology:

Advancements in imaging technologies, such as functional magnetic resonance imaging (fMRI) and positron emission tomography (PET), enable researchers to visualize and study the brain's response to pain. These insights contribute to a deeper understanding of pain perception and processing.

## Exploring Inflammatory and Immune Components:

Chronic pain often involves inflammatory responses and immune system interactions. Research endeavors focus on dissecting the roles of inflammatory molecules and immune cells in chronic pain conditions, paving the way for targeted anti-inflammatory therapies.

# Technological Advancements

## Transformative Tools for Pain Management:

Technological advancements play a pivotal role in shaping the landscape of chronic pain management, offering innovative tools and solutions to enhance treatment options.

## Wearable Devices and Biofeedback:

Wearable devices equipped with biosensors provide real-time data on physiological parameters. Biofeedback mechanisms empower individuals to monitor and modulate their physiological responses, contributing to self-regulation and pain management.

## Virtual Reality (VR) and Augmented Reality (AR):

VR and AR technologies offer immersive experiences that distract individuals from pain and create virtual environments conducive to relaxation. These technologies hold promise for managing acute and chronic pain, particularly during medical procedures or therapeutic interventions.

## Telehealth and Remote Monitoring:

The rise of telehealth facilitates remote consultations, enabling individuals to access healthcare professionals and pain management strategies from the comfort of their homes. Remote monitoring technologies enhance healthcare providers' ability to assess treatment effectiveness and adjust interventions as needed.

## Neuromodulation Devices:

Neuromodulation devices, including spinal cord stimulators and transcranial magnetic stimulation (TMS), deliver targeted electrical impulses to modulate neural activity. These devices offer a non-pharmacological approach to managing chronic pain by influencing pain signaling pathways.

# Hope for Future Treatments

## Promising Avenues for Relief:

As research and technology converge, the future of chronic pain management holds promising avenues for transformative treatments that aim to address the root causes of pain and enhance overall well-being.

## Precision Medicine Approaches:

The advent of precision medicine involves tailoring treatments based on individual characteristics, including genetic makeup, lifestyle, and environmental factors. Precision medicine holds the potential to optimize treatment outcomes by aligning interventions with the unique needs of each individual.

## Advanced Drug Therapies:

Ongoing research in pharmaceuticals explores novel drug therapies targeting specific pain receptors and pathways. From opioid alternatives to medications influencing immune responses, these innovations aim to provide effective pain relief with minimized side effects.

## Regenerative Medicine:

Emerging fields within regenerative medicine explore the potential of stem cell therapies and tissue engineering for repairing damaged tissues and mitigating the underlying causes of certain chronic pain conditions. These regenerative approaches offer a glimpse into future possibilities for long-term relief.

## Brain-Computer Interfaces (BCIs):

BCIs represent a cutting-edge intersection of neuroscience and technology. These interfaces enable direct communication between the brain and external devices, opening new possibilities for modulating pain perception and potentially rewiring neural pathways associated with chronic pain.

# Empowering Individuals through Knowledge

# Navigating the Ever-Evolving Landscape:

As we conclude our exploration of chronic pain management, it is essential to recognize the empowering role that knowledge plays in navigating the ever-evolving landscape of research and innovation.

## Informed Decision-Making:

Staying informed about current research, technological advancements, and emerging treatments empowers individuals to make informed decisions about their healthcare. Knowledge is a powerful tool that enhances advocacy for personalized and effective pain management strategies.

## Open Dialogue with Healthcare Providers:

Engaging in open and collaborative dialogues with healthcare providers fosters a partnership in navigating available treatments and exploring emerging options. Communication ensures that individuals actively participate in shaping their pain management plans.

## Participation in Clinical Trials:

For those seeking cutting-edge treatments, participation in clinical trials contributes to the advancement of medical knowledge and provides access to novel interventions. Clinical trials offer individuals the opportunity to be at the forefront of innovative therapies.

## Cultivating Hope and Resilience:

While the journey of chronic pain management involves challenges, cultivating hope and resilience remains paramount. The advancements in research and technology underscore a commitment to improving the lives of individuals with chronic pain, instilling optimism for the future.